WORKBOOK

SEX TRAPS

Dr. Wanda Davis-Turner

Take note that the name satan and related names are not capitalized. We choose not to acknowledge him, even to the point of violating grammatical rules.

Treasure House
An Imprint of
Destiny Image® Publishers, Inc.
P.O. Box 310
Shippensburg, PA 17257-0310

"For where your treasure is,
there will your heart be also." Matthew 6:21

ISBN 1-56043-300-0

For Worldwide Distribution
Printed in the U.S.A.

Second Printing: 2002   Third Printing: 2002

This book and all other Destiny Image, Revival Press, MercyPlace, Fresh Bread, Destiny Image Fiction, and Treasure House books are available at Christian bookstores and distributors worldwide.

For a U.S. bookstore nearest you, **call 1-800-722-6774**.
For more information on foreign distributors, **call 717-532-3040**.
Or reach us on the Internet: **www.destinyimage.com**

DEDICATION

I wish to dedicate this workbook to the most supportive people in my life, my family. In all my years, God has highly honored me to have parents, brothers, and sisters who have loved me, affirmed the call of God on my life, and united as a "clan" in support of my ministry to men, women, boys, and girls caught in sex traps.

My parents: Bishop Lewis D. and Mrs. Mary M. Stallworth.
My sisters: D. Marilyn, Dorthy, Gayle, Carole, and Dollye.
My brothers: Lewis, David, Richard, Neal, John, Mark, and Will Allen.

To them I say, "Thanks for your loyalty, thanks for encouraging the video, book, and now workbook for the ministry of *Sex Traps*."

ACKNOWLEDGMENTS

I am grateful to the Staff Publisher of Treasure House, Elizabeth C. Allen, and her associates for their dedicated assistance in completing this project. Additionally, I wish to thank my very special "brother-in-love," Reverend Michael Loyd, for his support and editorial assistance.

CONTENTS

How to Use This Study Guide

This study guide is designed for both individual growth and for group interaction. Questions are divided in three sections for each chapter. Materials needed include the following: your Bible; *Sex Traps*; this accompanying study guide; a small notebook for private answers; a pencil or pen; a blackboard or dry erase board; chalk or dry erase markers.

The first section of each chapter serves as a review, a stimulus for understanding the ideas in *Sex Traps*. By answering these questions—which adhere closely to the text of each chapter—you will be required to examine the author's main points.

The next section requires your introspection and prayer. You are not expected to share your answers for this section; you may write them on a separate sheet of paper, notebook, or private diary if you prefer.

The final section is designed to promote discussion, to foster problem-solving. Work individually. Jot down your answers. If you are a leader of a large group, divide people into small groups. Select discussion leaders who will listen to the ideas verbally, then note main points on a blackboard or dry erase board—followed by a brainstorming/discussion session.

CHAPTER ONE

Wake Up, Your Passion Is on Fire!

1. What in particular does God say in Isaiah 57:20–58:1 to verify that it's time to expose and confront sex traps?

    _____

    _____

    _____

2. The bait that satan uses for sex traps is our own _____.

3. What are some good things passions can do, if used as God intended? Pick the best answer.
    a. birth nations, win wars
    b. seal marriages with unbreakable devotion
    c. rule our lives in every situation
    d. both a. and b.

4. If God created us to be a passionate people, if he has given us passion as a gift, then how can satan best use passion to put us in a sex trap? Pick the best answer.
    a. by twisting and distorting the truth
    b. by causing us to hate our sex partner and find another
    c. by arguing with our sex partner because we are dissatisfied
    d. by saying words that we will regret

5. What are some negative things passion can do when we are led astray by satan? Pick the best answer.
    a. destroy nations, ignite wars, bring violent death
    b. make obstacles impassable,
    c. destroy marriages
    d. all of the above

6. In John 10:10, what does Jesus give as the cure for sexual sin? _____

    _____

    _____

    _____

7. In exposing our sin, God wants an answer from us. He wants us to make a _____.

8. Our sex traps are holding us back from God's plans for us. He has a greater _____ and _____ for this earth.

Application to My Life:

Answer each of these questions privately, in a prayerful attitude. Confront the sex traps in your life. Honestly consider each of these questions or issues as they impact you.

9. Think about the passion in your life. What passionate feelings do you use to create "good"? _____
    _____
    _____
    _____

10. Our twisted, distorted passions lead us to bait hidden in the snare.
    a. What passions have become twisted in your life? _____
        _____
        _____
        _____

    b. How has giving in to these passions led to wrong choices in your life? _____
        _____
        _____
        _____

11. What specific ways have these wrong choices hurt yourself or others? _____
    _____
    _____
    _____

12. Consider God's words in Leviticus 26:1, 14-16. What are the idols that you have placed above God? ___
    _____
    _____
    _____
    _____

Small Group Application:

These questions can be answered individually, then shared with a small group for discussion, brainstorming, and problem-solving. Use the space below to jot down your ideas individually first.

SUGGESTION: Each person's ideas can be shared verbally to a group leader who writes them on a blackboard.

13. God desires to change dirty diapers from the pulpit to the pew. How would you approach the idea of discussing the danger of sex traps in your own church, expecially if the people always seem to push this subject under the rug? Be specific about what steps you would take. _____

_____

_____

_____

_____

_____

_____

_____

_____

14. Jot down what you would say to a Christian friend who has fallen headlong into a sex trap. Explain how our passions can work as God created them or can lure us into a sex trap. _____

_____

_____

_____

_____

_____

_____

_____

_____

15. What would you say or do if a Christian friend came to you for help to escape a sex trap? He says that he's been trying to escape and knows Jesus can help him. He has prayed but is sinking fast. _____

_____

_____

_____

_____

_____

CHAPTER TWO

Five Roads That Lead to Sex Traps

1. One definition of sex is "the intimate exchange of physical, emotional, and spiritual parts or properties with or without consent." How does this acceptable definition of sex reveal why so many Christians are held in bondage to sex traps? _____

    _____

    _____

    _____

    _____

2. Which statement is false? Some of the results of being snared in sex traps are:
    a. sexually transmitted diseases, unwanted pregnancy, years of counseling
    b. rising cost of welfare, increasing divorce rate, broken homes
    c. an awareness of who we are
    d. a generation seeking drugs, gangs, and promiscuity

3. Confusion about God's plan for sex and sexual desire has caused problems in the Body of Christ. Choose the best word to complete this sentence: We show this confusion when we present an indiscriminate release of....
    a. anger
    b. love
    c. sexual signals
    d. money

4. What is the bait for a sex trap that a room full of women—even Christian women—may take while they talk in a beauty parlor? _____

    _____

    _____

5. What was the bait that King David took before he sinned with Bathsheba? See Second Samuel 11:2.

    _____

    _____

    _____

6. True or false? Once a person is saved, that person does not have to worry about sex traps. Why or why not?

    _____

    _____

    _____

7. What remedy do we have to avoid the bait in the sex traps? See First John 2:16-17. _____

    _____

    _____

8. Two errors, or misconceptions, concerning how sex should be regarded have caused extensive damage to the the church during the past several hundred years. Pick these two misconceptions.
    a. Sex is dirty and unclean.
    b. Sex is something we must study.
    c. Real Christians aren't affected by sexual desire.
    d. Sexy songs are bad.

9. Someone who continually falls for the bait in the sex traps, continually loses control and wants more and more becomes a sex _____.

10. What are the five roads leading to sex traps? _____

    _____

    _____

    _____

    _____

11. Which of the five roads did Solomon take when he "loved many strange women"? (See I Kings 11:1-4.)

    _____

    _____

Application to My Life:

Answer each question individually.

12. Think about your own personality, your own desires. Which of the five roads leading to sex traps most easily attract you? Why? _____

    _____

    _____

    _____

    _____

13. Think of specific situations where you may have begun walking down one or more of these roads.
    a. How far did you continue on the road? What happened as you progressed? Are you now fully caught in the sex trap from your travel down this road? _____

    _____

    _____

_____

_____

b. Did you resist a walk down a particular road—or roads? What made you turn away to take a better path? What damage to your life have you prevented? _____

_____

_____

_____

_____

14. You never will be who you really can be until you acknowledge who God says you really are.
   a. Who does God tell you that you are to Him? (If you don't have a clue, spend some time praying, asking God to tell you. Read Psalm 139:14.) _____

_____

_____

_____

_____

   b. How does God's view of you differ from how you perceive yourself? _____

_____

_____

_____

_____

   c. How does God's view of you help you resist the bait, the roads, all the temptations leading to sex traps?

_____

_____

_____

_____

Small Group Application:

Complete the questions individually, then share in a small group.

15. Give specific examples of advertising that baits people into sex traps. What can you do in your own home so your family does not fall prey to these baits? _____

_____

_____

_____

_____

_____

_____

_____

_____

16. You are bothered by the bait a female singer gives each time she performs at your church. Her clothes and body language are suggestive. In light of the seriousness of sex traps, what would you do? _____

_____

_____

_____

_____

17. King David's wandering eyes caused him trouble. You are a church youth group leader, or maybe you have a couple of teenagers in your family. What do you advise teens who are going steady but constantly talking about other people who look "so fine"? _____

_____

_____

_____

_____

18. Look at the five roads leading to sex traps. From your observations of people depicted in the media, how are each of these five roads shown as good paths to take? Give specific examples of characters in movies and on television. _____

_____

_____

_____

_____

CHAPTER THREE

Traps, Trappers, and Trappees

1. The four powerful truths of Psalm 124:6-8 give us hope that we can be freed from the snares of sex. Use the space below to draw pictures showing what happens to the bird—which represents our souls—in each of four steps.

    a. _____

    b. _____

    c. _____

    d. _____

2. If the Lord has freed us from the traps, has freed our souls, then what responsibility do we have in making sure we stay out of the snares? Pick the best answer.
    a. find a steady mate
    b. go to counseling
    c. find a circle of friends
    d. free our bodies

3. Victims caught in sex traps eventually become _____, themselves.

4. Christians are vulnerable to the snares of a sex traps because they often don't know the _____they are in, and they don't know that God has provided an _____.

5. A trap may catch, hold, and hurt its victim but what is its ultimate purpose? _____
    _____

6. Bait lures the trappee to the trap. What drives the trappee to go after the bait?
    a. the desire for satisfaction of a need or want
    b. the feeling that he is superior
    c. the desire for a new job
    d. a book she has just read

7. When Solomon—in the seventh chapter of Proverbs—teaches a young man how to avoid the wiles of an adultress, he specifically advises the young man to seek _____ and _____.

8. Scan the chapter and identify some of the some major sex traps today. _____
_____
_____

9. Read Hebrews 13:4a for insight. Pick the best answer. The only protective sex is in:
   a. the use of birth control
   b. limitation of partners
   c. the use of birth control
   d. marriage

10. Any sexual activity outside of the marriage covenant is considered what? _____
_____

11. Our bondage in a sex trap starts with the first, lingering _____.

12. We may be a target of satan just because we are pastors with ministries. What advice does Jesus give us to help avoid being ensnared in a trap when you visit a person as part of your ministry? Read Mark 6:7.
_____
_____

13. Fill in the blanks for the formula for sin. Forbidden _____ + attractive _____ + _____ in secrecy = sin.

14. Explain how satan's deceit works to ensnare a victim in a sex trap. _____
_____
_____

15. When are we the most vulnerable to satan's setups? _____
_____
_____

Application to My Life:

Answer each question individually.

16. Imagine you see the bait of a sex trap. Make the situation something which may seem plausible to you. But, you are one step ahead of the trap and don't go for the bait. What would you, as the potential trappee, say to the trapper? Don't hold back. _____
_____
_____

_____

_____

_____

_____

_____

_____

17. If you are not sprung from a sex trap by someone—or by your own hands—the result will be the death of your dreams and vision. Consider the situation in question 16. As the potential trappee, what would you stand to lose if you gave in, allowing the teeth of the snare to grab you totally? Be specific.

_____

_____

_____

_____

_____

18. What are wounds in your own life that most likely would make you vulnerable to the bait of a sex trap?

_____

_____

_____

_____

19. Take these wounds to God and ask Him to heal the wounds, to sweep you away from any sex traps which may "seem" to heal these wounds. Visualize yourself as a sheep with the Good Shepherd. Read Jesus' words in John 10:3-5 and Psalm 23).

Small Group Application:

Complete the questions individually, then share in a small group.

20. Decide how you would explain each part of Psalm 124: 6-8 to a person who is tightly caught in a sexual snare. Jot down main points. Next, pair off in twos and role play, telling the other person how the advice in this Psalm can help him or her. Then, exchange roles. _____

_____

_____

_____

21. Someone you know has been worn down by a sex trap; she is a prostitute. She says that she has tried to change her life, but this is the only way to find self-worth. Apply Psalm 139:14 to the situation. What would you tell her? Is she the trapper or the trappee? _____

_____

_____

_____

_____

_____

_____

_____

_____

_____

_____

22. Based on this same Scripture, what would you tell a man who continually seeks out prostitutes? Is he the trapper or the trappee? _____

_____

_____

_____

_____

_____

23. What would you say to a young clergyman, or clergywoman, to explain that his/her ministry makes him/her a target of sex traps? The person does not believe you. Be convincing. Pair off and try your arguments on your partner. _____

_____

_____

_____

_____

_____

_____

_____

_____

CHAPTER FOUR

The Victims of Sex Traps

1. How does Genesis 2:23-24 confirm that spiritual bonding occurs during sexual intimacy? _____

    _____

    _____

    _____

    _____

2. Pick the best answer. The spiritual bonding that occurs from sexual intimacy within a sex trap will hurt us because:
    a. We lose our individuality.
    b. Our personality is not being true to who God says we are
    c. God intended spiritual bonding through sexual intimacy only to be through marriage.
    d. All of the above.

3. God stresses that we are to give ourselves physically in marriage. God created men to be _____ of women, not _____.

4. What was the highest price God paid to rid the world of sin? Pick the best answer.
    a. He had to flood the world.
    b. He was disappointed in his children.
    c. He gave his only begotten Son.
    d. Both a. and b.

5. Jesus Christ broke the circles of _____.

6. When religious hypocricy is mixed with the sin of sex traps, it not only hurts the victim but also causes the victim's _____ in God to be destroyed.

7. A prostitute, most likely, was a trappee before she became a trapper. Based on Jesus' reaction to the situation where the woman was caught in adultry, in the eighth chapter of John, what would He tell a church to say/do to a prostitute who came for help? Pick the best answer.
    a. Go away until we have proof that you have repented of your sins.
    b. Come to church but sit in the back and leave quickly.
    c. Repent and stop the prostitution.
    d. If she has repented, the congregation should take up the cross and help her.
    e. both c. and d.

8. Most of our serious sexual problems stem from deviations, failures, or problems in the _____ relationship.

9. Homosexuals were not born that way.
   a. Most likely, what was the homosexual's relationship to his mother and father? _____

   b. Homosexuals always will be incomplete until they do what? _____

      _____

      _____

10. What is a common way that lesbians set a sex trap among female church members? _____

    _____

    _____

    _____

    _____

    _____

    _____

11. As quoted from the book, *Desires in Conflict*, by Joe Dallas, what are the three desires that can overpower the sex trap of homosexuality or lesbianism? Pick the best answer.
    a. desire to fit in a church, desire to have friends, desire to seek counseling
    b. desire to love God, desire for normal sex life, desire to be transparent
    c. desire to find a permanent mate, desire to read about the problem, desire for family
    d. desire to relocate, desire to join church committees, desire to see the pastor

12. Explain why there is no quick fix for homosexuality—why the process to overcome this sex trap takes time. _____

    _____

    _____

    _____

    _____

    _____

13. Explain how making the connection between knowledge and understanding leads to making right judgments—a necessary step in overcoming homosexuality. _____

    _____

    _____

    _____

    _____

    _____

    _____

Application to My Life:

Answer each question individually.

14. What do you think Jesus would say to someone who is trapping children in a sexual snare? Consider Jesus' words in Matthew 18. _____

_____

_____

15. Think about your own childhood. Were you involved as the victim of a sex trap? If so, what steps can you take to free yourself from the teeth of the trap? _____

_____

_____

_____

16. What specific changes can you make in your life to avoid the hidden sex traps—to ensure that you will put God first in your life? _____

_____

_____

17. Do you know someone who is in the sex trap of homosexuality, lesbianism, prostitution? Pray about what you, as a Christian, should do to help that person. Apply what you read in this chapter. What would you say to that person? Write down specific actions you can take.

_____

_____

_____

_____

_____

_____

Small Group Application:

Complete the questions individually, then share in a small group.

18. A young person whom you have known for a long time has been the victim of a sex trap baited by a clergyman. The person, hurting and doubting God's love, comes to you. You may be a pastor yourself. How do you approach one of these "little ones," who not only was trapped but also is disillusioned by religious hypocrisy? _____

_____

_____

_____

19. You know the clergyman in the above question. What would you say to him about his role as a trapper? If he is truly repentant, should he stay in his position? _____

_____

_____

_____

_____

20. Your children want to watch a popular television show starring a lesbian or a homosexual. The sexual orientation and lifestyle are no secret in the weekly episodes. What do you say to your children? Will watching the show hurt your family? _____

_____

_____

_____

21. You son or daughter—in high school or college—has been baited continually by another classmate of the same sex. You have witnessed the advances while the classmate is in your home, but your child seems to be unaware of what is happening. Your child's response to your questioning is: "I don't know what you are talking about. This person is just my friend." What course do you take? _____

_____

_____

_____

_____

_____

22. Your husband has left his family and children to move in with another man. You and your children are devastated, and you are trying to put your lives back together. You try to keep the lines of communication open with your husband, as you hope he will use Jesus to escape this sex trap. One day, your apparently repentant husband wants to come home. What do you do?

_____

_____

_____

_____

_____

_____

_____

CHAPTER FIVE

It's the Bait That Seals Your Fate

1. Explain how bait in a sex trap is both deceit and an idol all rolled in one. _____

    _____

    _____

    _____

    _____

2. The key to escape a sex trap is not to struggle. Escape comes from _____. The real battleground is within your _____. (From the book, *Can You Stand to be Blessed?* by Bishop T.D. Jakes.)

3. The way to put God first is by making Him the one you _____ the first and the most.

4. Read Psalm 124:6-8. We are freed by the Lord but we need continual help from Him to destroy the broken snares. What some examples of broken sexual snares that keep enticing an escapee? _____

    _____

    _____

    _____

    _____

    _____

    _____

5. Pick the best answer. What step should you take if you find that you are resisting the sex traps but they still remain close to you?
    a. Hang around the traps and try to see what really happened to you.
    b. See if you can talk to the people who were trying to trap you.
    c. Move away from the traps, change locations.
    d. Test yourself—go to the traps and see if you can resist temptation.

6. The devil doesn't just want to hurt you. He is out for your _____.

7. Pick the best answer. In remembering "no ringy, no dingy," how does this apply to the women who continually share too much of their lives—houses and cars—with single men?
    a. A woman who becomes too involved in a man's life can become sexually intimate without marriage.
    b. A woman should hold out for the most expensive ring and all the fine things in life.
    c. A woman should become engaged, then have sex.
    d. both a and c.

Application to My Life:

Answer each question individually.

8. To resist the bait of sex traps, we must understand that we instinctly are attracted to what will fill our inner needs. What are some of your inner needs that may not be filled to your satisfaction? What can you do to meet these inner needs and avoid taking the sex trap bait? _____

_____

_____

_____

_____

9. Read Jude 20-25 to find keys to overcome the sex traps bait. What steps would you take to put this advice to work in your life? How would you reschedule your time to allow space to take these steps? _____

_____

_____

_____

_____

10. As Bishop T.D. Jakes says, the key to deliverance comes from within; the battleground of the mind is where victory comes. What are some of your recurring thoughts that may lead you to sex traps? For example, when you are tempted, do you tell yourself that you deserve a little fun? _____

_____

_____

_____

_____

Small Group Application:

Complete the questions individually, then share in a small group.

11. It's obvious that a friend who attends your church is baiting your pastor. You have talked to this friend, who denies anything is happening. She continues to be a trapper, setting the bait, and you see your pastor swaying. What do you do? _____

_____

_____

_____

_____

_____

12.   You are a clergyman who is being baited for a trap by an attractive, aggressive woman in your church. You have resisted but notice a growing attraction. What steps should you take to keep yourself from the snare?

_____

_____

_____

_____

_____

_____

13.   You are a young widow or widower who has many unfulfilled needs. Your friends constantly try to arrange "dates" with some very sexually aggressive men. After a few dates, you, as a Christian, know this feels wrong. How do you escape the bait? _____

_____

_____

_____

_____

_____

_____

CHAPTER SIX

The Direction of Your Desire Is Important

1. Since desire is God's gift to you, desire becomes evil when it is twisted by _____.

2. What are some of the lies satan is telling us about desire, lies that eventually come out of our own mouths? Pick the best answer.
   a. "Everybody is doing it."
   b. "If you love me, you will."
   c. "I really love you so you must..."
   d. "Did God really say we shouldn't....?"
   e. all of the above

3. Compare the lives of Joseph—who resisted temptation in Genesis 39—and Sampson who took the bait in Judges 16. Tell how the outcome of each of these men's lives was different because of the choices they made to take or resist the bait. _____

   _____

   _____

   _____

   _____

   _____

4. The attack by satan on godly masculinity is greater than ever.
   a. Why has satan picked the present time to attack godly masculinity? _____

   _____

   b. One of satan's most twisted attacks on man's natural instinct to protect children is_____.

   c. Later in life, what happens to children who are victimized by this, or other sex traps? _____

   _____

   d. Another attack on godly masculinity is _____.

5. Still another sex trap, which caught the pagans, is _____.

6. What does Proverbs 5:11 tell us about the wave of sexually transmitted diseases? _____

   _____

   _____

   _____

7. Joseph ran from Potiphar's wife. Explain how turning off the television can be compared to Joseph's escape. _____

_____

_____

_____

Application to My Life:

Answer each question individually.

8. Sampson's secret weakness caused him to fall into a sex trap. What are your secret weaknesses? Are they strong enough to cause your entrapment? How can you ensure that you won't be trapped? _____

_____

_____

_____

_____

9. Look to the advice of how to break away from satan, at the bottom of page 80 and top of page 81 of *Sex Traps*. If you now find yourself in the teeth of a sex trap, read these words and pray for deliverance. If you have resisted a sex trap but know a specific person who is ensnared, what would you add to these words?

_____

_____

_____

_____

10. If you presently are ensnared in a trap, take Joseph's lead—run! What steps do you intend to take in following his example? _____

_____

_____

_____

_____

11. Think of the things you desire the most. List them, then number them in order of importance. Which of these will lead you to God's plan for you? Which ones may lead to sex traps? _____

_____

_____

_____

_____

Small Group Application:

Complete the questions individually, then share in a small group.

12. List what you think are some of the "not so secret" weaknesses of today's world. How are these weaknesses applauded as strengths? _____

_____

_____

_____

_____

_____

13. What would you tell a young man who has been taught that he never should reveal weaknesses, just cover them up? What points would you make to him to show that surrendering to those weaknesses leads to sex traps? _____

_____

_____

_____

_____

14. Explain the danger of sex traps to a young lady who makes it her job to flirt with every man who crosses her path. _____

_____

_____

_____

_____

15. Consider how desire plays into the lives of people you know—even people in the limelight, celebrities, or government leaders. Give real examples of ways people use desire to create good. How does desire leading to sex traps destroy people's lives? _____

_____

_____

_____

_____

_____

CHAPTER SEVEN

The Deception That Leads to Death

1. The situation is set—the trap, the bait, the trappee, the twisted desire. All that's missing is deception. Explain how deception figures into the sex trap. Pick the best answer.
    a. Deception, as satan's messenger, whispers lies.
    b. Deception tells us what we want to hear so we can continue sinning.
    c. Deception to others is something you must use to get out of the trap.
    d. both a. and b.

2. Write down the formula for death as a mathematical equation as explained in Mike Murdock's book, *Winners*.

    _____ + _____ (leads to) _____ = _____.

3. How does your remembrance that God is watching at all times wipe out the lies of deception? _____

    _____

    _____

    _____

4. A homosexual, lesbian—or even a prostitute—are told lies by satan.
    a. What are these lies?

    _____

    _____

    _____

    b. What should a person already in one of these sex traps tell himself or herself in response to these lies?

    _____

    _____

    _____

    c. Once a person has confronted the deception, has repented, and has turned his/her life around, what is the next deception satan throws his/her way? Solomon was confronted with this deception in 1Kings 5:3-5.

    _____

    _____

    _____

5. Pick the best answer. What is the real death caused by being ensnared in a sex trap?
    a. the twisting of your mind
    b. separation from God
    c. sexually transmitted diseases
    d. loss of dignity

6. Repentance needs to be _____ and _____.

7. How do preachers fall into the trap of "I'm entitled" to my desire? _____

    _____

    _____

    _____

Application to My Life:

Answer each question individually.

8. If you are a someone who has escaped a sex trap and has repented, what does it mean to you that the evidence of your repentance must last a lifetime and touch your heart in the deepest places? _____

    _____

    _____

9. There is a measure to help you decide if an action you are taking is sinful or not. Is the action acceptable in Jesus' eyes? Think of your sexual sins that you would not want Jesus, the Good Shepherd, to see. How do you intend to change these actions? _____

    _____

    _____

    _____

    _____

    _____

10. If you have fallen into a sex trap and want to escape—or want to help another escape—read Second Corinthians 5:17.
    a. Ask God to make you a new person. Describe the new person you visualize. _____

    _____

    _____

    _____

    _____

    _____

    b. What would you say to satan to confirm that you are not what he says you are? See bottom of page 90 but think of your own emphatic words. _____

    _____

    _____

    _____

    _____

Small Group Application:

Complete the questions individually, then share in a small group.

11. Review Dr. Tony Evans' five truths about sexual sins. Put yourself in the situation of addressing a church group about sex traps. The people may not accept that they even need to hear about this topic. Explain each truth in one emphatic sentence to drive the message home. Choose your words carefully. Be creative!

_____

_____

_____

_____

_____

_____

_____

_____

12. Think about the real death, separation from the presence of God.
    a. When a person is caught in a sex trap, he strays from God. What are common actions people take to replace this lacking intimacy with God? _____

_____

_____

_____

_____

_____

    b. What are the characteristics of a person who is very close to God, with no separation? _____

_____

_____

_____

_____

_____

_____

CHAPTER EIGHT

Catch Me, But When You Do...Take Me to Jesus!

1. Why do people caught in sex traps often want to get caught? Pick the best answer.
   a. Drawing others into the sin is fun.
   b. They like to brag about what they do sexually.
   c. The heaviness of their sin has become unbearable.
   d. They want others to see that it's not their fault.

2. What must a person clenched in a sex trap surrender to Jesus to be set free? Pick the best answer.
   a. everything—including addictions, attractions, cravings
   b. more of his time to go to church functions
   c. all R-rated movies
   d. her desire to find the perfect person to marry

3. You can be assured that faith in Jesus will save you. God has compassion for the_____, the_____, and the truly _____ people of God who want out of their sex traps.

4. Read John 8: 1-11.
   a. What was the important message, the life direction, that Jesus gave to the woman caught in adultry?

   _____

   b. Why didn't He just forgive her—and send her down the road? _____

   _____

5. Consider the accusing people crowding around the woman.
   a. What did Jesus tell them? _____

   _____

   b. What advice is He giving us today when we catch someone in a sex trap?

   _____

   _____

   c. What is good advice for you to do before you begin to condemn someone caught in a snare?

   _____

6. God sees you as someone special.
   a. God reminds you that you are_____ in his household.
   b. You are royal_____because you have been bought with_____.
   c. Many of our problems arise because we don't know_____.

7. Reconsider the guideline that will help you stay away from sex traps: "Don't do anything that you don't want your_____ to see."

Application to My Life:

Answer each question individually.

8. Are you in a sex trap today? Have you ever thought about being caught? What relief will come with being caught, exposing your sin, and repenting? _____

_____

_____

_____

_____

_____

9. What, in particular, do you need to surrender to give up the sin of the sex trap? _____

_____

_____

_____

_____

_____

10. What will God give you to replace the sinful things that you have surrendered to Him? _____

_____

_____

_____

_____

_____

11. A sex trap will hinder you from reaching the destiny that God has planned for you. Pray sincerely. What is God's plan for you? How can you begin to follow the path to that plan? _____

_____

_____

_____

_____

_____

_____

Small Group Application:

Complete the questions individually, then share in a small group.

12. If you are the person catching someone in a sex trap, you may be considered the enemy. Keeping questions 8, 9, and 10 in mind, what would you say to the trappee to convince him or her that you are out to help? Be encouraging but firm. _____

_____

_____

_____

_____

13. Discuss a situation where you are a young man among friends who constantly brag about visiting prostitutes. You are belittled or called "gay" because you do not join them. What actions would you take? What would you say to your friends who are caught tightly in a sex trap? _____

_____

_____

_____

_____

_____

14. Your sister, a married Christian woman, is falling into a sex trap with a married man. So far, she has reached the point of having private lunches and long telephone conversations. Do you think the situation is serious enough to approach her about the trap? If so, what do you say or do? _____

_____

_____

_____

_____

_____

15. You try to help a friend, male or female, to escape a sex trap. Your friend has engaged in several sexual relationships within the past year. Presently, this friend is engaged in a sexual relationship outside of marriage. He/she already has seen a counselor—who encourages your friend to continue the relationship if he/she feels happy and fulfilled. What is your course of action? _____

_____

_____

_____

_____

_____

CHAPTER NINE

Rescue by Repentance, Not Resolution

1. It's not enough to say, "I'm never going to do this again."
   a. Explain why this statement will not help someone escape a sex trap. _____

   _____

   _____

   _____

   b. Resolution is merely your assertion that you will _____.

   c. Repentance is admitting your sin, expressing godly sorrow, then not _____ the sin.

2. Jesus says in Luke 9:23-26 that you should take up your cross daily and follow Him.
   a. Explain in your own words what Jesus means. _____

   _____

   _____

   _____

   _____

   b. Explain how taking up your cross is connected to repentance. _____

   _____

   _____

   _____

   _____

   c. The key to stop taking the bait of sex traps is to stop living the life that _____
   and start living the life that _____.

3. Romans 8:13-14 gives us keys to living the life which will ensure that we do not return to the old sex trap. Also see Romans 8:5-6. What are these keys? Pick the best answer.
   a. Do not live after the flesh or you will die.
   b. Live in the Spirit.
   c. Living in the Spirit will kill the sins of the flesh.
   d. Living in the Spirit will make you sons of God.
   e. All of the above.

4. Your only path to survival when you are caught in a sex trap is to _____.

5.   Explain what it means that God will meet you where you are. How does this truth apply to sex traps?

_____

_____

_____

_____

_____

_____

_____

Application to My Life:

Answer each question individually.

6.   Read Proverbs 6: 23-35 where Solomon gives advice on how to stay away from the sex trap of adultry.
   a.   Explain how keeping your eyes on Jesus will keep your eyes from straying to a person other than your husband or wife. _____

_____

_____

_____

_____

   b.   Think about your life. Be honest. If you find your eyes straying to another man or woman what are the first few steps you can take to fight this sex trap? _____

_____

_____

_____

_____

   c.   Have you ever thought you were the object of someone's straying eyes? What, if any, of your actions may be contributing to someone else's sex trap? If you honestly feel that you are not baiting the sex trap, what can you do about the situation? _____

_____

_____

_____

_____

7. If you are involved in a sex trap now—whether as a trapper or a trappee—and want to escape, pray with all your heart and ask God to help you. Now, write down the plan of action you will take to pull the teeth of the trap from your life. _____

    _____

    _____

    _____

    _____

    _____

    _____

8. If you have just repented of the sin of a sex trap, what will you do to ensure that you will not fall back into the trap? Be very specific about what actions you will take—how your life will change. _____

    _____

    _____

    _____

    _____

    _____

    _____

    _____

Small Group Application:

Complete the questions individually, then share in a small group.

9. Consider Jesus' reaction to the woman caught in adultry. Now consider the situation where your pastor has been caught in adultry. After talking with him, you believe his repentance is for real. A large group of people in your congregation want the pastor to leave the church immediately. What do you think? Will you get involved? Why or why not? If so, what will you do? _____

    _____

    _____

    _____

    _____

    _____

10. When you are in a battle to remove someone from a sex trap, whether it be yourself or another person, your real fight is with satan. Read Ephesians 6:12. Explain what putting on the armor means, especially to fight a sex trap. _____

_____

_____

_____

_____

_____

_____

11. You know a person who vows not to take the bait anymore because she fears sexually transmitted diseases. This person tells you that what she did is not a sin; it was "finding herself." What do you tell her about the importance of repentance, the worthlessness of resolutions without repentance? _____

_____

_____

_____

_____

_____

_____

_____

12. A co-worker confesses that he has led a homosexual lifestyle for the past five years. He has been praying and going to counseling. His homosexual friends—and the counselor—all tell him that he was born that way. Therefore, they say, repentance is not an issue. He is confused and asking for help. How do you lead him in the right direction? _____

_____

_____

_____

_____

_____

_____

_____

13. The youth leader in your church tells you that she once was a teen runaway who became a prostitute many years ago. This person shared her testimony of how she repented and gave up that lifestyle. You have a teen son and daughter in the youth group. Describe your feelings. Will you allow your children to continue in the group? What do you say to the leader after she shares her story? _____

_____

_____

_____

_____

_____

_____

_____

_____

_____

14. You are a young person who once was a trappee, a victim of a sex trap. You have escaped with the help of God. What steps do you take so that you do not become a trapper later in life? _____

_____

_____

_____

_____

_____

_____

_____

_____

_____

CHAPTER TEN

The Four "D's" of Deliverance

1. Let's emphasize what the four D's mean. Though simple, these words are so important to someone recovering from the wounds of a sex trap. Use your own words, your own definitions.

   a. What does "don't" mean? Consider how a child interprets this word when a parents says it.

   _____

   _____

   b. What does "don't do" mean?

   _____

   c. The meaning of "that" depends on the situation. Substitute "involve yourself in sex traps." Now, what does "don't do that" mean? _____

   _____

   _____

   d. Add the last word, "dummy." What is a dummy? _____

   _____

   _____

2. If you have escaped the jaws of a sex trap, why is it important to remind yourself about the "dummy" part of the four D's? Pick the best answer.

   a. In the flesh, you are a dummy. When you are talking to flesh, you need to remember that.
   b. Once you have escaped, you're immune from ever going back into the trap. "Dummy" just reminds you.
   c. Dummy is a term of endearment to yourself, to remind you that you're immune to sex traps now.
   d. You have been a dummy once and can be a dummy again by falling for another trap. Don't forget!
   e. both a. and d.

3. What makes us travel back to the broken pieces of our discarded sex trap? Pick the best answer.

   a. We feel the rush of emotions, the hunger of the flesh.
   b. We go back to try to see if we can tempt ourselves, which helps us to understand ourselves.
   c. We need to see the broken pieces, talk to the person who trapped—us which helps us overcome.
   d. Visiting the broken traps is good for us to show how brave we are now that we've escaped.

4. Read Second Peter 1:3-4. What will keep us from picking up those broken snares and putting them back together? _____

   _____

   _____

   _____

   _____

5. Remember, when the broken traps lie scattered all around us and we can't move them, the best advice is to_____.

6. Remember, Jesus Christ will help you if you receive Him into your heart. Read John 16:13. Who did Jesus say that He would send to help us avoid those broken snares? _____.

7. In First Corinthians 10:5-13, the apostle Paul tells you about escaping the rubbish of broken snares. God is faithful. He will not allow you to _____ a temptation longer than you are _____.

8. God will free you. However, what is your responsibility? _____

    _____

    _____

Application to My Life:

Answer each question individually.

9. Whether you are a trapper, a trappee, or someone who has never fallen in to a sex trap, thoughtfully take to heart the freedom prayer on pages 123 and 124.
    a. Do you give God "permission to break those sex ties"? _____
    b. Why is this an important step?

        _____

        _____

        _____

        _____

        _____

        _____

    c. When you say, "Sever me from my history," what part of your history do you mean?

        _____

        _____

        _____

        _____

    d. Picture that "precious blood of Jesus" washing over your mind, your whole body. Do you feel clean? Are you a new creature? How is your forgiveness connected to this blood? _____

        _____

        _____

        _____

        _____

        _____

e. Allow Jesus to take total "control of your memory." What painful memories are you giving to Him?

_____

_____

_____

_____

_____

_____

_____

f. Grab onto that "right spirit" that you asked the Lord to "renew" within you. Take some time. Truly listen to the Lord. Move only when and where He says. What does Jesus tell you about your next moves?

_____

_____

_____

_____

_____

_____

_____

g. Thank the Lord! You are free! Spend some time just "feeling" what freedom has done to you. Do you feel differently than you did a few moments ago? Describe your feelings. (Repeat the process until you break the sex trap bondage.)

_____

_____

_____

_____

_____

_____

_____

10. After saying the freedom prayer with meaning, think about "who" you really are in God's eyes. Ask God to reveal to you His plan for your life. What is your destiny? _____

_____

_____

_____

_____

_____

11. Reading the Bible and praying are two necessary parts of our lives if we are to discover what the "divine nature" is. For you, what amount of time do you need to spend on each of these? What are the main problems hindering you? How can you reorganize your days so you have time with the Lord? _____

_____

_____

_____

_____

_____

_____

_____

Small Group Application:

Complete the questions individually, then share in a small group.

12. Remember that satan has designed sex traps to destroy us, to demolish God's purpose for us. Look at the familiar paths created by God (see page 120). Jot down a few words to explain how sex traps destroy each path.

_____

_____

_____

_____

_____

_____

_____

_____

_____

_____

13. What activities—or—people do you think that we should fill our lives with—if we are trying to follow each of these paths as God intended? _____

_____

_____

_____

_____

_____
_____
_____
_____
_____

14. Now apply what you've learned. Imagine you are speaking to a group of teens. What would you tell them about sex traps in five minutes or less? Jot down ideas, then number them in order of importance.

_____
_____
_____
_____
_____
_____
_____
_____
_____
_____
_____
_____

15. You are a young person who has committed himself or herself to no sex before marriage. What do you say to encourage yourself to stay on the right course? How would you encourage a friend to follow God's way?

_____
_____
_____
_____
_____
_____
_____
_____
_____
_____

Answer Key

Chapter One: Wake Up, Your Passion Is on Fire!

1. "Shout it aloud, do not hold back. Raise your voice like a trumpet. Declare to My people their rebellion...."
2. passions
3. d.
4. a.
5. d.
6. He is the Way. "I am come that they might have life, and that they might have it more abundantly."
7. choice, decision
8. agenda ... plan
9. personalized response
10. a. and b. personalized response
11. personalized response
12. personalized response
13. personalized response shared with small group
14. personalized response shared with small group
15. personalized response shared with small group

Chapter Two: Five Roads That Lead to Sex Traps

1. desire for "intimate" exchange, which we substitute with sex, without regard for whether this exchange is "with" or "without" consent
2. c.
3. c.
4. surrendering to the temptation to talk with loose tongues, to tell too many sexual details of their marriages
5. what a man sees with his wandering eyes
6. false. Temptation affects all of us because we all are human.
7. do the will of God and not follow the way of the world
8. a. and c.
9. addict
10. desire for the forbidden, ego fulfullment, the world's pressure, the lie that you must reward yourself, and the fleshly craving for variety
11. craving for variety
12. personalized response
13. a. and b. personalized response
14. a., b., c. personalized response
15. personalized response shared with small group
16. personalized response shared with small group
17. personalized response shared with small group
18. personalized response shared with small group

Chapter Three: Traps, Trappers, and Trappees

1. a., b., c., and d. Suggested drawings: show God protecting soul, in shape of bird; show a bird escaping a snare; show a snare broken in pieces; show a bird flying high with God above.
2. d.
3. trappers
4. danger...escape
5. to destroy the victim
6. a.
7. wisdom...understanding
8. adultry, pornography, prostitution, homosexuality

9. d.
10. fornication, adultery, or perversion
11. look
12. go two by two, take another person with you
13. appetite...temptation...opportunity
14. to blind, confuse, or hide the truth
15. when you are wounded and hurting
16. personalized response
17. personalized response
18. personalized response
19. personalized response
20. personalized response shared with small group
21. personalized response shared with small group
22. personalized response shared with small group
23. personalized response shared with small group

Chapter Four: The *Victims* of Sex Traps

1. they shall be of one flesh, one body
2. d.
3. protectors...predators
4. c.
5. destruction
6. faith
7. e.
8. parent-child
9. a. Male figure likely hurt or disappointed the child; mother likely dominated the child.
    b. Repent and ask God to heal the pain within.
10. Sometimes, lesbians actively recruit sexual partners by acting as Christian advisors, then lay traps for heterosexual women.
11. b.
12. Homosexuality is symptomatic of other problems; universal sin is the real problem; faith in Christ is only the beginning; the person must fight to escape the snare.
13. Knowledge provides understanding, and understanding motivates us to make right judgments.
14. personalized response
15. personalized response
16. personalized response
17. personalized response
18. personalized response shared with small group
19. personalized response shared with small group
20. personalized response shared with small group
21. personalized response shared with small group
22. personalized response shared with small group

Chapter Five: It's the Bait That Seals Your Fate

1. Bait is enticement leading from freedom to bondage, a trick, a deception. Bait also is an idol, something you put before God; you disobey God by taking the bait, which is a sin.
2. within...mind
3. love
4. addictions, old habits, temptations from trappers, freshened bait
5. c.
6. life
7. a.
8. personalized response

9. personalized response
10. personalized response
11. personalized response shared with small group
12. personalized response shared with small group
13. personalized response shared with small group

Chapter Six: The Direction of Your Desire Is Important

1. deceit
2. e.
3. When Joseph ran from the bait, he was unjustly punished for a time. God later rewarded him with a promotion. Sampson took the bait which was a means to cut his hair and take his strength—which was a gift from God. Joseph's outcome was better.
4. a. These are the endtimes.
    b. pedophilia
    c. Victims become trappers later in life.
    d. homosexuality
5. bestiality
6. Sex traps destroy the body, a temple to God.
7. Certain shows on television provide bait—similar to the bait of Potiphar's wife. One look leads to another and eventually to being ensnared.
8. personalized response
9. personalized response
10. personalized response
11. personalized response
12. personalized response shared with small group
13. personalized response shared with small group
14. personalized response shared with small group
15. personalized response shared with small group

Chapter Seven: The Deception That Leads to Death

1. d.
2. desire + deception (leads to) disobedience = death
3. Following through with an action based on deception does not hold up under the Savior's steady gaze.
4. a. "You were born this way." "You can't change what you want." "You need this thing that you desire."
    b. God is not homosexual, or lesbian, or a prostitute. Since He created me in His image, I do not have to take on this label.
    c. "Now you deserve a reward for all you've endured."
5. b.
6. lifelong...heart-deep
7. It's similar to Solomon's attitude: "The King Am I."
8. personalized response
9. personalized response
10. a. and b. personalized response
11. personalized response shared with small group
12. a. and b. personalized response shared with small group

Chapter Eight: Catch Me, But When You Do...Take Me to Jesus!

1. c.
2. a.
3. lost...hurting...hungry
4. a. Repent and sin no more.
    b. She needed to know that her fight was not over; she had to resist temptation.
5. a. Whoever is without sin, cast the first stone.
    b. We are all sinners so don't condemn. Help the person, instead.
    c. Switch places with the one in the sex trap.

6. a. royalty
    b. seed...blood
    c. who we are in Christ
7. Savior
8. personalized resoponse
9. personalized response
10. personalized response
11. personalized response
12. personalized response shared with small group
13. personalized response shared with small group
14. personalized response shared with small group
15. personalized response shared with small group

Chapter Nine: Rescue by Repentance, Not Resolution

1. a. Your own strength will not ensure that we won't fall into the trap again.
    b. quit something
    c. repeating
2. a. You must resist temptation every day to stop the sin of the sex trap; this struggle to resist becomes your cross.
    b. True repentance brings forgiveness from Jesus and gives you the ability to stop taking the bait of a sex trap. But, the cross you carry, the struggle, will be with you.
    c. We want to live...God wants us to live.
3. e.
4. Pray from the heart.
5. God requires repentance, a surrendered life. Then, he will continue the healing work by starting at the point of where you are in your life; He will bring restoration to your life if you let Him.
6. a., b., and c. personalized response
7. personalized response
8. personalized response
9. personalized response shared with small group
10. personalized response shared with small group
11. personalized response shared with small group
12. personalized response shared with small group
13. personalized response shared with small group
14. personalized response shared with small group

Chapter Ten: The Four "D's" of Deliverance

1. a. "no"
    b. "Do not take a particular course of action"
    c. "Don't take the bait; don't go for the sex trap!"
    d. one who is stupid
2. e.
3. a.
4. partaking of the divine power of God so that we take on a divine nature
5. Move away from the broken traps, change locations.
6. the Holy Spirit
7. suffer...able
8. to stay free
9. a., b., c., d., e., f., and g. personalized response
10. personalized response
11. personalized response
12. personalized response shared with small group
13. personalized response shared with small group
14. personalized response shared with small group
15. personalized response shared with group

Exciting titles
by Dr. Wanda Turner

▬ SEX TRAPS

Discover the tactics of the enemy that lead you down the road of unparalleled remorse. Satan's traps are set with a burning desire to birth pain, guilt, and shame in your life. Learn to avoid the traps!
ISBN 1-56043-193-8

▬ *Also available as a workbook.*
ISBN 1-56043-300-0

▬ CELEBRATE CHANGE

Celebrate Change is for people of all ages and circumstances who want to learn to transform the "pain of change" into the "celebration of change": Think of your faith as a spiritual muscle and change as the machine that exercises your faith. Celebrating change is an act of our will. It cannot occur until we accept change, and that requires the work of God through the Holy Spirit. Dr. Turner's life-story is poignant, relevant and encouraging.
ISBN 0-7684-3031-3

▬ BEHIND THE POWER

For too long, we have ignored the wives of powerful men. They are seen as well-dressed, pampered insignificant accessories to their husbands' success. They are seldom credited with contributing to their husbands' prosperity and too often blamed when it falters. *Behind the Power* gives honor where it is due, gives light where there is little understanding, and tools to help today's wives live full and fulfilled lives.
ISBN: 0-7684-3032-1

▬ I STOOD IN THE FLAMES

If you have ever come to a point of depression, fear, or defeat, then you need this book! With honesty, truth, and clarity, Dr. Turner shares her hard-won principles for victory in the midst of the fire. You can turn satan's attack into a platform of strength and laughter!
ISBN 1-56043-275-6

Don't miss any one of these exciting videos by Dr. Wanda Turner.
These messages can change your life!

SEX TRAPS
1 video   ISBN 0-7684-0030-9

PRIVATE DELIVERANCE IN A PUBLIC PLACE
1 video   ISBN 0-7684-0054-6

REMEMBER TO FORGET
1 video   ISBN 0-7684-0048-1

THE OTHER MIRACLE
1 video   ISBN 0-7684-0053-8

GOD'S ORIGINAL PLAN FOR THE FAMILY
1 video   ISBN 0-7684-0049-X

Available at your local Christian bookstore.

**For more information and sample chapters,
visit www.destinyimage.com**

6B-2:7